Achieving Excellence in Manufacturing through Robotic Process Automation An Engineer's Perspective

Jakob

1

Copyright © [2023]

Author: Jakob

Title: Achieving Excellence in Manufacturing through Robotic Process Automation An Engineer's Perspective

This book is a product of [Publisher's Jakob]

ISBN:

TABLE OF CONTENTS

Chapter 1: Introduction to Robotic Process Automation in Manufacturing

Understanding the Role of Automation in Manufacturing

Automation has revolutionized the manufacturing industry, allowing companies to streamline their processes, improve productivity, and achieve higher levels of efficiency. In recent years, the concept of Robotic Process Automation (RPA) has gained significant traction, offering engineers a powerful tool to achieve excellence in manufacturing.

RPA involves the use of software robots or bots to automate repetitive and rule-based tasks within a manufacturing process. These bots can perform a wide range of activities, such as data entry, inventory management, quality control, and even complex decision-making processes. By taking over these tasks, RPA frees up human workers to focus on more value-added activities, such as innovation, problem-solving, and customer interaction.

One of the key benefits of RPA in manufacturing is its ability to enhance accuracy and precision. Unlike humans, robots do not suffer from fatigue, distractions, or errors due to inconsistencies in performing repetitive tasks. This not only ensures consistent quality in products but also minimizes the risk of defects and rework, ultimately saving time and costs.

Moreover, RPA enables manufacturers to achieve higher levels of productivity and efficiency. Bots can work 24/7 without breaks, leading to increased output and reduced cycle times. They can also handle multiple tasks simultaneously, enabling parallel processing and eliminating bottlenecks in the production line. As a result, manufacturers can meet customer demands faster, reduce lead times, and gain a competitive edge in the market.

Additionally, RPA promotes flexibility and adaptability in manufacturing processes. With the ability to reprogram and reconfigure bots, engineers can easily modify production lines to accommodate changes in product design, volume, or customer requirements. This agility allows manufacturers to respond quickly to market fluctuations, optimize resource allocation, and improve overall operational performance.

However, it is important for engineers to understand that RPA is not a replacement for human workers but rather a tool to augment their capabilities. While robots can perform repetitive tasks with precision, they lack the creativity, problem-solving skills, and emotional intelligence that humans possess. Therefore, it is crucial for engineers to identify the right balance between human and robotic involvement in manufacturing processes, ensuring that humans are still at the forefront of critical decision-making and complex problem-solving tasks.

In conclusion, the role of automation, particularly Robotic Process Automation, in manufacturing cannot be underestimated. It offers engineers the opportunity to achieve excellence in manufacturing by enhancing accuracy, productivity, efficiency, and flexibility. By leveraging RPA, engineers can optimize their operational processes, reduce costs, and deliver high-quality products to meet customer expectations.

Overview of Robotic Process Automation (RPA)

Robotic Process Automation (RPA) has emerged as a game-changing technology in the field of manufacturing. This subchapter provides an in-depth overview of RPA, its key concepts, and the benefits it offers to engineers working in the niche of Robotic Process Automation.

RPA refers to the use of software robots or artificial intelligence (AI) to automate repetitive, rule-based tasks in manufacturing processes. These robots are capable of mimicking human actions, interacting with digital systems, and executing tasks with precision and efficiency. By automating such tasks, engineers can focus on more complex and value-added activities.

One of the key advantages of RPA is its ability to improve operational efficiency. By automating routine tasks, engineers can eliminate errors caused by human intervention and reduce the time required to complete them. This allows for faster and more accurate processing, leading to increased productivity and cost savings. Moreover, RPA enables engineers to handle high-volume tasks without the need for additional manpower.

Another significant benefit of RPA is its impact on quality control. With its ability to execute tasks consistently and accurately, RPA minimizes the risk of human errors, ensuring consistent quality across the manufacturing process. Engineers can leverage RPA to implement robust quality assurance mechanisms, resulting in improved product quality and customer satisfaction.

Furthermore, RPA enhances flexibility and scalability in manufacturing operations. As the demands of the market change, engineers can easily reconfigure RPA systems to adapt to new requirements. This allows for faster response times and increased agility in meeting customer needs. Additionally, RPA enables engineers to scale up or down operations without significant disruptions, making it an invaluable tool for managing fluctuating production volumes.

When implementing RPA, engineers should consider the potential impact on the workforce. While RPA can automate repetitive tasks, it does not replace human workers. Instead, it frees up their time to focus on more complex and creative aspects of their roles. Engineers should proactively engage with the workforce, providing training and upskilling opportunities to ensure a smooth transition and maximize the benefits of RPA.

In conclusion, RPA holds immense potential for engineers working in the niche of Robotic Process Automation. By automating repetitive tasks, RPA improves operational efficiency, enhances quality control, and enables flexibility in manufacturing processes. However, successful implementation requires careful consideration of the workforce and effective change management strategies. With RPA, engineers can achieve excellence in manufacturing and drive innovation in the industry.

Benefits of RPA in Manufacturing

In today's rapidly evolving world, the manufacturing industry is continuously seeking ways to stay ahead of the competition and streamline their operations. One revolutionary technology that has emerged as a game-changer is Robotic Process Automation (RPA). In this subchapter, we will explore the numerous benefits that RPA brings to the manufacturing sector, specifically addressing engineers and those interested in Robotic Process Automation.

Increased Efficiency and Productivity: One of the primary advantages of integrating RPA into the manufacturing process is the significant increase in efficiency and productivity. By automating repetitive and mundane tasks, engineers can focus their valuable time and expertise on more complex and strategic activities. RPA eliminates the need for manual data entry, reduces errors, and accelerates the overall production process. This increased efficiency leads to improved productivity, reduced lead times, and enhanced customer satisfaction.

Cost Reduction: Implementing RPA in manufacturing can result in substantial cost savings. By automating tasks that were previously carried out manually, manufacturers can reduce labor costs and reallocate resources to more value-added areas. RPA also minimizes the risk of human error, leading to fewer production mistakes and associated costs. Additionally, RPA can optimize inventory management, reducing the need for excess stock and minimizing storage costs.

Enhanced Quality Control: In the manufacturing industry, maintaining high-quality standards is crucial. RPA plays a vital role in ensuring consistent quality control by performing repetitive tasks with precision and accuracy. By automating quality checks, RPA eliminates the potential for human error and ensures that each product meets the required specifications. This leads to improved product quality, reduced defects, and ultimately, higher customer satisfaction.

Improved   Safety:
Safety is a paramount concern in manufacturing, and RPA can contribute to a safer working environment. By automating hazardous tasks or those involving heavy machinery, RPA reduces the risk of accidents and injuries. Engineers can program robots to perform dangerous tasks, such as handling toxic chemicals or operating in high-temperature environments, thus protecting human workers from potential harm.

Flexibility   and   Scalability:
RPA offers manufacturers the flexibility to adapt to changing market demands and scale their operations accordingly. Robots can be easily reprogrammed and redeployed to accommodate new product lines or variations. This agility allows manufacturers to respond quickly to market trends and customer demands, thereby gaining a competitive edge.

In conclusion, the benefits of RPA in manufacturing are significant and diverse. From increased efficiency and productivity to cost reduction, enhanced quality control, improved safety, and flexibility, RPA has the potential to revolutionize the manufacturing industry. As engineers and enthusiasts of Robotic Process Automation, it is crucial to embrace this technology and explore its full potential in achieving excellence in manufacturing.

Challenges and Limitations of RPA in Manufacturing

As engineers dive into the world of Robotic Process Automation (RPA) in the manufacturing industry, it is important to understand the challenges and limitations associated with this technology. While RPA offers numerous benefits, it is not without its share of obstacles that need to be addressed for successful implementation.

One of the primary challenges engineers face when implementing RPA in manufacturing is the complexity of processes. Manufacturing operations involve a wide range of tasks, from simple repetitive actions to complex decision-making processes. RPA is best suited for automating repetitive and rule-based tasks, but when it comes to more intricate processes requiring human judgment and decision-making, RPA may fall short. Engineers must carefully analyze the processes they aim to automate and identify the limitations of RPA in handling such tasks.

Another challenge is the integration of RPA systems with existing manufacturing systems and technologies. Many manufacturing facilities already have an array of legacy systems in place that may not be compatible with RPA. Engineers need to ensure seamless integration between RPA and existing systems, which often requires additional time and effort.

Additionally, RPA implementation in manufacturing often requires a significant amount of data handling. RPA relies on accurate and up-to-date data to perform tasks efficiently. However, manufacturing environments may have data scattered across various systems and databases, making it difficult to ensure data integrity and accessibility for RPA solutions. Engineers must develop robust data management strategies to overcome this challenge and ensure that RPA systems have access to the required data.

Furthermore, cybersecurity is a critical concern when implementing RPA in manufacturing. As RPA systems interact with sensitive manufacturing data and control systems, they become potential targets for cyberattacks. Engineers must implement robust security measures to protect against unauthorized access, data breaches, and other cybersecurity threats.

Lastly, resistance to change and lack of employee acceptance can hinder the successful implementation of RPA in manufacturing. Some employees may fear that RPA will replace their jobs, leading to resistance and reluctance to embrace the technology. Engineers must address these concerns through effective communication and employee training programs to ensure a smooth transition and maximize the benefits of RPA.

In summary, while RPA holds immense potential for transforming manufacturing processes, engineers must be aware of the challenges and limitations associated with its implementation. By understanding and addressing these challenges, engineers can overcome obstacles and leverage RPA to achieve excellence in manufacturing.

Scope and Objectives of the Book

In the rapidly evolving field of manufacturing, embracing technological advancements is crucial to stay ahead of the competition. Robotic Process Automation (RPA) has emerged as a game-changer, offering immense potential to improve efficiency, productivity, and quality in manufacturing operations. This book, titled "Achieving Excellence in Manufacturing through Robotic Process Automation: An Engineer's Perspective," aims to provide engineers in the niche of Robotic Process Automation with a comprehensive guide to understanding, implementing, and optimizing RPA in manufacturing processes.

The scope of this book is to equip engineers with the knowledge and tools necessary to leverage the power of RPA in manufacturing. It covers a wide range of topics, starting with an introduction to RPA and its applications in the manufacturing industry. The book delves into the technical aspects of RPA, including programming languages, software platforms, and hardware requirements, giving readers a solid foundation to build upon.

Furthermore, this book explores the various challenges and considerations associated with implementing RPA in a manufacturing environment. It addresses concerns such as integration with existing systems, data security, and workforce implications. By understanding these challenges, engineers can proactively plan and strategize for a successful RPA implementation.

One of the key objectives of this book is to provide practical insights into the best practices for RPA implementation. It offers real-world case studies and examples that illustrate how RPA has been successfully applied in different manufacturing scenarios. Readers will gain valuable insights into the potential benefits, limitations, and risks associated with RPA, enabling them to make informed decisions when implementing automation solutions.

Additionally, this book aims to foster a mindset of continuous improvement and innovation among engineers. It discusses emerging trends and technologies in RPA, such as machine learning, artificial intelligence, and Internet of Things (IoT), and their potential impact on manufacturing processes. By staying updated on the latest advancements, engineers can proactively identify opportunities for further optimization and automation in their manufacturing operations.

In conclusion, "Achieving Excellence in Manufacturing through Robotic Process Automation: An Engineer's Perspective" serves as a comprehensive guide for engineers in the niche of Robotic Process Automation in the manufacturing industry. It covers the scope of RPA, from its technical aspects to implementation challenges and best practices. By reading this book, engineers can unlock the potential of RPA, enhance their understanding of automation technologies, and drive excellence in manufacturing operations.

Chapter 2: Fundamentals of Robotic Process Automation

Definition and Evolution of RPA

In recent years, the field of Robotic Process Automation (RPA) has gained significant attention and interest in the manufacturing industry. RPA refers to the use of software robots or artificial intelligence to automate repetitive and rule-based tasks that were previously performed by humans. These tasks can range from data entry and processing to invoice generation and order tracking. The primary goal of RPA is to enhance operational efficiency, reduce costs, and improve accuracy in manufacturing processes.

At its core, RPA is a technology that enables the creation of virtual workers or software robots that mimic human actions and interact with various applications and systems. These robots can perform tasks with precision and speed, without the need for human intervention. RPA leverages technologies such as machine learning, natural language processing, and artificial intelligence to automate complex tasks that were once thought to be exclusively within the realm of human capabilities.

The evolution of RPA can be traced back to the early 2000s when it was primarily used in the banking and financial sectors. However, with advancements in technology and the increasing demand for process automation, RPA has found its way into the manufacturing industry. Today, RPA is being implemented in various manufacturing processes, including supply chain management, inventory control, quality assurance, and production scheduling.

One of the key benefits of RPA in manufacturing is the ability to streamline workflows and reduce manual errors. By automating repetitive tasks, engineers can focus their efforts on more complex and strategic activities, leading to increased productivity and improved decision-making. RPA also enables real-time data collection and analysis, providing engineers with valuable insights into process performance and identifying areas for improvement.

Another significant advantage of RPA is its scalability and flexibility. RPA solutions can be easily modified and adapted to changing business requirements, allowing manufacturers to quickly respond to market dynamics and optimize their operations. Additionally, RPA can integrate with existing IT systems, eliminating the need for extensive infrastructure changes and reducing implementation time and costs.

As the manufacturing industry continues to embrace automation and digital transformation, RPA is poised to play a crucial role in achieving excellence in manufacturing. Engineers, as the driving force behind process improvement and innovation, need to understand the potential of RPA and its applications in their respective niches. By leveraging RPA, engineers can revolutionize manufacturing processes, enhance competitiveness, and pave the way for a more efficient and sustainable future.

Key Components of RPA Systems

In the rapidly evolving field of Robotic Process Automation (RPA), engineers play a crucial role in designing and implementing efficient systems that can revolutionize manufacturing processes. To achieve excellence in manufacturing through RPA, it is crucial to understand the key components that make up these systems. This subchapter aims to provide engineers with an in-depth understanding of the essential elements of RPA systems.

1.   Robotic   Process   Automation   Software: At the heart of any RPA system lies the software that enables automation. This software is designed to mimic human actions, such as data entry, data extraction, and decision-making processes. Engineers must choose the right RPA software that aligns with the specific manufacturing requirements and integrates seamlessly with existing systems.

2.   Artificial   Intelligence   and   Machine   Learning: To enhance the capabilities of RPA systems, engineers often incorporate artificial intelligence (AI) and machine learning algorithms. These technologies enable the automation software to learn from patterns, make intelligent decisions, and adapt to changing conditions. Engineers need to understand AI and machine learning concepts to harness the full potential of RPA systems.

3.   Process   Mapping   and   Design: Before implementing RPA, engineers need to analyze existing manufacturing processes and identify potential areas for automation. Process mapping and design involve documenting the current workflow, identifying bottlenecks, and optimizing the process for

automation. This step ensures that the RPA system is tailored to the specific needs of the manufacturing environment.

4.   Robotic   Hardware:
In some cases, RPA systems may require physical robots or robotic arms to perform tasks that cannot be accomplished solely through software automation. Engineers must select the appropriate robotic hardware based on factors such as payload capacity, reach, and precision. Integrating hardware with the software ensures a seamless automation process.

5.   Data   Integration   and   Security:
RPA systems heavily rely on data from various sources within the manufacturing environment. Engineers must ensure that the RPA system can integrate with different data sources, such as ERP systems, databases, and sensors. Additionally, data security measures must be implemented to protect sensitive information and prevent unauthorized access.

6.   Monitoring   and   Analytics:
To continuously improve the efficiency and effectiveness of RPA systems, engineers need to monitor their performance and gather relevant data. Analytics tools can provide insights into system performance, identify areas for improvement, and enable proactive maintenance. Engineers should design monitoring mechanisms to ensure optimal performance and identify potential issues in real-time.

In conclusion, understanding the key components of RPA systems is essential for engineers aiming to achieve excellence in manufacturing through automation. By leveraging the right software, incorporating AI and machine learning, mapping processes, selecting appropriate hardware, integrating data securely, and implementing monitoring and analytics, engineers can design and implement RPA systems that optimize manufacturing processes and drive efficiency in the industry.

Types of Robots Used in Manufacturing

In the rapidly evolving field of manufacturing, robots have emerged as indispensable tools for enhancing efficiency, precision, and productivity. Their ability to perform repetitive tasks with great accuracy and speed has revolutionized the industry, making them an integral part of any modern manufacturing facility. This subchapter aims to provide engineers with a comprehensive overview of the various types of robots commonly used in manufacturing processes, highlighting their unique capabilities and applications.

1. Industrial Robots: These versatile robots are designed to handle heavy payloads and perform a wide range of tasks, such as material handling, welding, assembly, and painting. They are typically equipped with multiple axes of motion, allowing for complex and precise movements. Industrial robots are known for their high reliability and repeatability, making them ideal for mass production and high-speed applications.

2. Collaborative Robots (Cobots): Unlike traditional industrial robots, cobots are designed to work alongside human operators, promoting a collaborative and safe working environment. Cobots are equipped with advanced sensors and force feedback technology, allowing them to detect and respond to human presence, ensuring human-robot interaction is safe and efficient. These robots are commonly used in assembly lines, quality control, and small-scale production.

3. Mobile Robots: As the name suggests, mobile robots are designed to move autonomously within a manufacturing facility. They are equipped with navigation systems, such as lasers or cameras, enabling them to navigate complex environments and avoid obstacles. Mobile robots are particularly useful in material handling, logistics, and

inventory management, as they can transport goods efficiently and seamlessly across different parts of the facility.

4. SCARA Robots: SCARA (Selective Compliance Articulated Robot Arm) robots are widely used in assembly and pick-and-place applications. They have a horizontal arm that moves in a planar motion, allowing for fast and precise movements. SCARA robots are known for their high-speed performance, making them suitable for applications that require rapid and accurate positioning.

5. Delta Robots: These robots are characterized by their unique design, with three arms connected to a common base, forming a triangular shape. Delta robots are commonly used in high-speed pick-and-place applications, particularly in the food and packaging industries. Their lightweight design and fast movements make them ideal for tasks that require quick and precise handling.

By understanding the different types of robots used in manufacturing, engineers can make informed decisions when selecting the most suitable robot for a specific application. Each type of robot offers distinct advantages and capabilities, allowing manufacturers to automate processes and achieve higher levels of efficiency, accuracy, and productivity. As the field of robotic process automation continues to advance, engineers must stay updated with the latest developments and leverage the potential of these remarkable machines to achieve excellence in manufacturing.

Integration of RPA with Existing Manufacturing Systems

In recent years, Robotic Process Automation (RPA) has emerged as a game-changing technology in the manufacturing industry. RPA offers a unique opportunity to streamline operations, optimize processes, and achieve excellence in manufacturing. For engineers working in the field of Robotic Process Automation, understanding the seamless integration of RPA with existing manufacturing systems is crucial.

The integration of RPA with existing manufacturing systems presents numerous benefits for engineers and the manufacturing industry as a whole. By automating repetitive and manual tasks, RPA reduces human error, increases productivity, and enhances overall efficiency. It allows engineers to focus on more complex and value-adding activities, thus accelerating innovation and improving the quality of products.

To successfully integrate RPA with existing manufacturing systems, engineers must consider several key factors. Firstly, a thorough understanding of the existing systems and their processes is essential. This includes identifying areas where RPA can have the greatest impact and analyzing the compatibility of RPA with the current infrastructure.

Next, engineers need to evaluate the scalability and flexibility of the RPA solution. Manufacturing systems often undergo changes and updates, so the chosen RPA platform must be adaptable to meet evolving requirements. This ensures that the integration remains effective in the long run.

Another crucial aspect is data management. RPA relies on accurate and real-time data to perform tasks. Engineers must establish reliable data sources and implement robust data collection and analysis mechanisms. This ensures that the RPA system operates efficiently and produces reliable results.

Furthermore, engineers should consider the security implications of integrating RPA with existing manufacturing systems. As RPA interacts with sensitive data and controls critical processes, a strong security framework must be implemented to safeguard against potential cyber threats and unauthorized access.

Collaboration among different stakeholders is also vital for successful integration. Engineers should work closely with IT departments, operations teams, and management to ensure seamless integration and address any challenges that may arise during the process.

In conclusion, the integration of RPA with existing manufacturing systems holds great potential for engineers and the manufacturing industry. By automating repetitive tasks, improving efficiency, and enhancing data management, RPA can revolutionize manufacturing processes. However, successful integration requires careful planning, evaluation of scalability, robust data management, and collaboration among stakeholders. With a well-executed integration strategy, engineers can achieve excellence in manufacturing through Robotic Process Automation.

Ensuring Data Security and Privacy in RPA

In today's rapidly evolving technological landscape, Robotic Process Automation (RPA) is revolutionizing the manufacturing industry, offering engineers unprecedented opportunities to enhance productivity and streamline operations. As engineers delve into the realm of RPA, it is crucial to understand and address the paramount concerns of data security and privacy.

Data security is a top priority when implementing RPA in manufacturing processes. With the increasing reliance on interconnected systems and the vast amounts of data being processed, engineers must be vigilant in safeguarding sensitive information. This subchapter aims to equip engineers in the niche of Robotic Process Automation with the knowledge and tools necessary to ensure data security and privacy.

To begin with, it is essential to identify potential vulnerabilities in the RPA system. Engineers must conduct a comprehensive risk assessment to identify areas where data breaches or unauthorized access may occur. By analyzing the entire process, from data collection to storage and transmission, engineers can proactively identify and mitigate potential risks.

Implementing robust authentication and access control mechanisms is another critical aspect of data security. Engineers must ensure that only authorized personnel can access sensitive data and that strong passwords and multi-factor authentication methods are in place. Additionally, encryption techniques should be employed to protect data both at rest and in transit, mitigating the risk of unauthorized interception.

Regular monitoring and auditing of the RPA system are essential to identifying any potential security breaches promptly. Engineers should establish a system that continuously monitors network traffic, logs activities, and promptly alerts any suspicious behavior. By conducting periodic security audits, engineers can identify vulnerabilities and implement necessary updates or patches.

Furthermore, privacy concerns must be addressed to maintain compliance with relevant regulations and standards. Engineers should understand the legal and regulatory requirements specific to their industry and ensure that the RPA system adheres to these guidelines. Anonymization and pseudonymization techniques can be employed to protect personally identifiable information and maintain privacy.

Lastly, engineers must prioritize data backup and disaster recovery plans. Regularly backing up data and having a robust disaster recovery strategy in place ensures that critical information is not lost in the event of a system failure, cyberattack, or natural disaster.

In conclusion, as engineers explore the realm of Robotic Process Automation in manufacturing, data security and privacy must be at the forefront of their considerations. By conducting risk assessments, implementing robust authentication and access control measures, monitoring and auditing the system, adhering to privacy regulations, and prioritizing data backup and disaster recovery, engineers can ensure the safe and secure implementation of RPA in their processes. With a solid foundation in data security and privacy, engineers can achieve excellence in manufacturing through Robotic Process Automation.

Chapter 3: Applications of RPA in Manufacturing Processes

RPA in Material Handling and Warehousing

In recent years, Robotic Process Automation (RPA) has emerged as a game-changing technology in the field of manufacturing. With its ability to automate repetitive and mundane tasks, RPA has revolutionized various industries, including material handling and warehousing. In this subchapter, we will explore the impact of RPA in material handling and warehousing, focusing on its benefits, applications, and challenges.

One of the key advantages of RPA in material handling and warehousing is its ability to enhance operational efficiency. By automating tasks such as inventory management, order picking, and packaging, RPA reduces the likelihood of errors and improves overall productivity. This not only saves time but also reduces costs associated with manual labor. Engineers can design and implement RPA systems to optimize processes and streamline operations, leading to improved throughput and increased customer satisfaction.

RPA also plays a crucial role in ensuring the accuracy and reliability of material handling and warehousing operations. With its advanced algorithms and machine learning capabilities, RPA can analyze vast amounts of data in real-time, enabling engineers to make data-driven decisions. This not only minimizes the risk of human error but also allows for proactive maintenance and optimization of equipment, leading to improved overall equipment effectiveness (OEE).

Furthermore, RPA enables engineers to deploy smart and flexible robots that can adapt to changing requirements in material handling and warehousing. These robots can collaborate with human workers, augmenting their capabilities and improving safety. By automating repetitive and physically demanding tasks, RPA reduces the risk of injuries and frees up human workers to focus on more complex and value-added activities.

However, implementing RPA in material handling and warehousing is not without its challenges. Engineers need to carefully analyze the existing processes and design RPA systems that seamlessly integrate with the existing infrastructure. They must also consider factors such as scalability, security, and compatibility with other automation technologies.

In conclusion, RPA has the potential to revolutionize material handling and warehousing operations. By automating repetitive tasks, improving operational efficiency, and enhancing overall accuracy and reliability, RPA enables engineers to achieve excellence in manufacturing. However, successful implementation requires careful planning, collaboration, and a deep understanding of the specific requirements of the material handling and warehousing industry.

RPA in Assembly and Production Lines

As the manufacturing industry continues to evolve and embrace automation, Robotic Process Automation (RPA) has emerged as a game-changing technology for optimizing assembly and production lines. RPA, also known as software robotics, offers a myriad of benefits to engineers working in the niche of Robotic Process Automation.

One of the key advantages of RPA in assembly and production lines is its ability to enhance efficiency and productivity. By automating repetitive and rule-based tasks, engineers can free up valuable time to focus on more complex and value-added activities. RPA robots can perform tasks with extreme accuracy and precision, reducing the risk of human error and ensuring consistent quality throughout the manufacturing process.

Moreover, RPA can significantly improve the speed of assembly and production lines. Robots equipped with RPA software can execute tasks at a much faster rate than humans, leading to increased output and shorter cycle times. This increased speed not only improves overall productivity but also allows manufacturers to meet tight deadlines and customer demands more effectively.

Another crucial aspect that engineers should consider is the flexibility provided by RPA in assembly and production lines. RPA robots can be easily programmed and reprogrammed to adapt to changing manufacturing requirements. This flexibility allows for rapid adjustments to accommodate product variations, customization, or changes in the assembly process. Engineers can leverage RPA to create agile production lines that can quickly respond to market demands and ensure optimal resource utilization.

Additionally, RPA offers significant cost savings for manufacturers. By automating tasks that were previously performed by human workers, companies can reduce labor costs and minimize the risk of workplace injuries. Furthermore, RPA robots can operate 24/7 without the need for breaks or shifts, leading to enhanced production efficiency and higher overall equipment effectiveness.

However, engineers must also be aware of the challenges and considerations associated with implementing RPA in assembly and production lines. The successful integration of RPA requires careful planning, process mapping, and collaboration between engineers and RPA experts. Ensuring compatibility between existing systems, training employees on RPA usage, and addressing potential security concerns are all crucial steps to achieve a seamless and efficient RPA implementation.

In conclusion, RPA has the potential to revolutionize assembly and production lines, providing engineers with a powerful tool to optimize processes, improve productivity, and drive manufacturing excellence. By embracing RPA, engineers in the niche of Robotic Process Automation can achieve higher levels of efficiency, quality, and cost-effectiveness, ultimately contributing to the success of their organizations in the dynamic manufacturing landscape.

RPA in Quality Control and Inspection

In the fast-paced world of manufacturing, ensuring product quality and maintaining high inspection standards are critical. The rise of Robotic Process Automation (RPA) has revolutionized quality control and inspection processes, providing engineers with innovative solutions to achieve excellence in manufacturing.

RPA, a technology that uses software robots or "bots" to automate repetitive tasks, has found its niche in quality control and inspection. These bots are capable of performing a wide range of tasks, from data collection and analysis to product testing and evaluation, with unparalleled speed and accuracy.

One of the primary advantages of RPA in quality control is its ability to eliminate human errors. Traditional inspection processes often rely on manual labor, which is prone to mistakes and inconsistencies. With RPA, engineers can leverage advanced algorithms and machine learning capabilities to ensure consistent and error-free inspections. Bots can be programmed to follow specific inspection protocols, detecting even the slightest deviations from the desired standards, thus significantly reducing the risk of defective products reaching the market.

Furthermore, RPA can streamline the data collection and analysis process, saving engineers valuable time and resources. Bots can be programmed to gather data from various sources, such as sensors, databases, and even external systems, and perform real-time analysis. This enables engineers to make informed decisions promptly, leading to quicker problem-solving and improved overall quality control.

Another key benefit of RPA in quality control is its scalability. As manufacturing processes evolve and production volumes increase, RPA can easily adapt and accommodate growing demands. Engineers can deploy additional bots or modify existing ones to handle higher workloads, ensuring consistent and efficient quality control and inspection across the manufacturing floor.

It is worth mentioning that RPA does not replace human involvement but rather enhances it. Engineers can focus on higher-value tasks, such as process optimization, innovation, and continuous improvement, while bots handle the repetitive and mundane inspection activities. This collaboration between humans and robots enables manufacturers to achieve excellence in manufacturing by leveraging the best of both worlds.

In conclusion, RPA has emerged as a game-changer in quality control and inspection for engineers in the field of Robotic Process Automation. By automating repetitive tasks, eliminating human errors, streamlining data collection and analysis, and offering scalability, RPA empowers engineers to achieve excellence in manufacturing. With RPA as a powerful tool in their arsenal, engineers can ensure consistent product quality, meet stringent inspection standards, and drive innovation in the manufacturing industry.

RPA in Inventory and Supply Chain Management

In today's fast-paced world of manufacturing, inventory and supply chain management play a crucial role in ensuring seamless operations and customer satisfaction. However, manual processes often lead to inefficiencies, errors, and delays. This is where Robotic Process Automation (RPA) comes into play, offering engineers in the field of Robotic Process Automation a powerful tool to revolutionize inventory and supply chain management.

RPA can automate various tasks involved in inventory and supply chain management, streamlining processes and improving overall efficiency. One of the key benefits of RPA is its ability to handle repetitive and time-consuming tasks with precision and speed. For instance, RPA bots can be programmed to automatically update inventory levels, generate purchase orders, and track shipments, eliminating the need for manual intervention. By automating these tasks, engineers can save valuable time and redirect their efforts towards more strategic activities.

Furthermore, RPA can enhance inventory accuracy by minimizing human errors and discrepancies. With RPA bots, engineers can ensure real-time tracking of inventory, reducing the risk of stockouts or overstock situations. By constantly monitoring inventory levels and generating alerts when thresholds are reached, RPA enables proactive decision-making, preventing potential disruptions in the supply chain.

Additionally, RPA can seamlessly integrate with existing software systems, such as Enterprise Resource Planning (ERP) or Warehouse Management Systems (WMS), creating a unified platform for inventory and supply chain management. This integration enables data synchronization across different departments and facilitates real-time visibility into inventory levels, order status, and delivery timelines. By providing accurate and up-to-date information, RPA empowers engineers to make informed decisions, optimize inventory levels, and implement lean manufacturing practices.

Another significant advantage of RPA in inventory and supply chain management is its scalability. As manufacturing operations grow or change, RPA can adapt and scale effortlessly to accommodate evolving needs. Whether it is handling increased order volumes during peak seasons or integrating new suppliers into the supply chain, RPA can flexibly adjust to meet the demands of the business, ensuring uninterrupted operations and customer satisfaction.

In conclusion, RPA offers engineers in the field of Robotic Process Automation a powerful tool to enhance inventory and supply chain management. By automating repetitive tasks, improving accuracy, enabling real-time visibility, and providing scalability, RPA revolutionizes the way manufacturing organizations manage their inventory and supply chain processes. Embracing RPA in this domain can lead to increased operational efficiency, reduced costs, and improved customer satisfaction, making it an indispensable tool for engineers aiming to achieve excellence in manufacturing.

RPA in Maintenance and Predictive Analytics

In recent years, Robotic Process Automation (RPA) has revolutionized the manufacturing industry by streamlining various processes and enhancing overall efficiency. However, its impact on maintenance and predictive analytics is often overlooked. In this subchapter, we will explore the role of RPA in maintenance and how it can significantly contribute to achieving excellence in manufacturing.

Maintenance in manufacturing facilities is crucial to ensure uninterrupted operations and prevent costly breakdowns. Traditionally, maintenance tasks have been performed manually, leading to potential delays and errors. With RPA, engineers can automate routine maintenance activities, such as equipment inspections, data collection, and preventive maintenance scheduling. By deploying robots to perform these tasks, engineers can focus their expertise on more critical and complex maintenance activities, ultimately improving the overall reliability and availability of manufacturing systems.

Furthermore, RPA can be integrated with predictive analytics to enhance maintenance strategies. Predictive analytics leverages historical data, real-time monitoring, and machine learning algorithms to predict equipment failures and optimize maintenance schedules. By combining RPA with predictive analytics, engineers can automate the data collection and analysis process, enabling proactive maintenance actions. This integration enables a more data-driven approach to maintenance, reducing downtime, and increasing productivity.

One key advantage of RPA in maintenance is its ability to collect and analyze large volumes of data quickly and accurately. Robots can be programmed to gather data from various sources, such as sensors, production systems, and maintenance logs, ensuring that all relevant information is captured for analysis. Additionally, robots can perform complex data analysis tasks, identifying patterns and anomalies that might go unnoticed by humans. This enables engineers to make informed decisions based on reliable data, leading to more effective maintenance strategies.

Moreover, RPA can facilitate remote maintenance and troubleshooting, especially in large-scale manufacturing facilities or geographically dispersed sites. By deploying robots equipped with cameras and sensors, engineers can remotely inspect and diagnose equipment issues, eliminating the need for physical presence. This not only saves time and resources but also enables faster response times, minimizing production losses.

In conclusion, RPA is a game-changer in the field of maintenance and predictive analytics. By automating routine tasks, integrating with predictive analytics, and enabling remote maintenance, RPA empowers engineers to achieve excellence in manufacturing. As engineers, it is essential to embrace RPA and explore its potential in optimizing maintenance strategies, improving reliability, and driving overall operational excellence.

Chapter 4: Implementing RPA in Manufacturing

Assessing the Feasibility and ROI of RPA Implementation

Introduction:

In today's rapidly evolving manufacturing industry, engineers are constantly seeking innovative ways to optimize processes and streamline operations. Robotic Process Automation (RPA) has emerged as a game-changing technology that offers tremendous potential to achieve excellence in manufacturing. However, before diving into RPA implementation, it is crucial for engineers to assess the feasibility and Return on Investment (ROI) of such a transformation. This subchapter aims to guide engineers through the process of evaluating the feasibility and ROI of RPA implementation in manufacturing, helping them make informed decisions.

Understanding   Feasibility:

Feasibility analysis plays a pivotal role in determining whether RPA implementation is viable within the manufacturing environment. Engineers must thoroughly assess various factors such as process complexity, system compatibility, data availability, and resource requirements. By conducting a comprehensive feasibility study, engineers can identify potential challenges and limitations, helping them plan the implementation process more effectively.

Evaluating   ROI:

Return on Investment (ROI) is a crucial metric that determines the financial viability and success of any automation initiative. Engineers need to quantify the potential benefits of RPA implementation, including increased productivity, reduced errors, improved quality, and enhanced customer satisfaction. By conducting a thorough cost-benefit analysis, engineers can calculate the ROI and effectively communicate the potential advantages to key stakeholders.

Factors Affecting Feasibility and ROI: Several factors influence the feasibility and ROI of RPA implementation in manufacturing. These include process complexity, data security requirements, system integration challenges, and regulatory compliance. Engineers need to consider these factors while evaluating the feasibility and ROI, ensuring they align with the strategic goals and objectives of the organization.

Risk Assessment: Implementing RPA in manufacturing involves inherent risks, such as system failures, data breaches, and resistance to change. Engineers must conduct a comprehensive risk assessment to identify potential risks and develop mitigation strategies. By addressing risks proactively, engineers can minimize disruptions and ensure a smooth transition towards RPA implementation.

Conclusion:
Assessing the feasibility and ROI of RPA implementation is a critical step for engineers aiming to achieve excellence in manufacturing through automation. By thoroughly evaluating factors like process complexity, system compatibility, and data availability, engineers can determine the feasibility of RPA implementation. Additionally, conducting a cost-benefit analysis and risk assessment enables engineers to quantify the potential ROI and minimize associated risks. This subchapter equips engineers with the necessary knowledge and tools to make informed decisions about RPA implementation, empowering them to drive efficiency, productivity, and success within

the niches of Robotic Process Automation in the manufacturing
sector.

39

Identifying Suitable Processes for RPA

When it comes to implementing Robotic Process Automation (RPA) in manufacturing, engineers play a critical role in identifying suitable processes that can be automated. This subchapter aims to provide engineers with a comprehensive understanding of how to identify the right processes for RPA, ensuring optimal efficiency and productivity gains in the manufacturing environment.

The first step in identifying suitable processes for RPA is to conduct a thorough analysis of the existing manufacturing processes. Engineers need to evaluate the complexity, repetitiveness, and rule-based nature of each process. Processes that are highly repetitive, rules-driven, and involve a significant number of manual tasks are ideal candidates for automation through RPA. By automating these processes, engineers can eliminate human errors, reduce cycle times, and improve overall process quality.

Another important factor to consider when identifying suitable processes for RPA is the potential return on investment (ROI). Engineers need to assess the financial impact of automating a particular process. This involves analyzing the cost savings, increased productivity, and reduced operational risks that RPA can bring. By prioritizing processes with a high ROI, engineers can ensure that the implementation of RPA delivers the desired benefits to the manufacturing organization.

Furthermore, engineers should also consider the scalability and flexibility of the processes. It is crucial to choose processes that can easily adapt to changes in the manufacturing environment. RPA solutions should be able to accommodate variations in product specifications, volumes, and production schedules without significant reprogramming efforts. This flexibility ensures that the automation remains effective in the long run and can be expanded to other areas of the manufacturing process.

Additionally, engineers should collaborate closely with the end-users and other stakeholders to identify pain points and bottlenecks in the manufacturing processes. By understanding the challenges faced by the workforce on the shop floor, engineers can prioritize processes that will have the most significant impact on improving efficiency and job satisfaction. Involving end-users in the decision-making process will also increase acceptance and adoption of RPA within the organization.

In conclusion, identifying suitable processes for RPA is a crucial step towards achieving excellence in manufacturing through automation. Engineers need to evaluate the complexity, repetitiveness, and rule-based nature of each process, assess the ROI, consider scalability and flexibility, and collaborate with end-users. By following these guidelines, engineers can successfully implement RPA, leading to enhanced productivity, reduced costs, and improved quality in the manufacturing environment.

Designing and Developing RPA Solutions

In the rapidly evolving field of Robotic Process Automation (RPA), engineers play a pivotal role in creating innovative solutions that revolutionize manufacturing processes. This subchapter delves into the intricacies of designing and developing RPA solutions, providing engineers with invaluable insights and practical guidance to achieve excellence in this domain.

The first step in designing an RPA solution is to thoroughly understand the manufacturing process and identify areas where automation can bring about significant improvements. Engineers need to closely collaborate with stakeholders, including production managers and operators, to gain a comprehensive understanding of the existing workflow and potential pain points. This invaluable knowledge serves as the foundation for developing an effective RPA solution.

Once the problem areas are identified, engineers can begin the process of designing the RPA solution. This involves mapping out the desired automation flow, defining the tasks and activities that the robots will perform, and determining the optimal sequence of actions. Engineers need to carefully analyze the feasibility and potential challenges associated with each step, ensuring that the RPA solution is efficient, reliable, and scalable.

Furthermore, engineers must consider the technical aspects of developing RPA solutions. They need to select the appropriate automation tools and technologies that align with the specific requirements of the manufacturing process. This may involve leveraging machine learning algorithms, natural language processing, or computer vision to enable robots to interact intelligently with humans and their environment.

Testing and validation are crucial steps in the development process. Engineers must rigorously test the RPA solution to ensure its functionality, accuracy, and stability. This involves conducting extensive simulations, running pilot programs, and collecting feedback from operators. Iterative improvements and fine-tuning are essential to optimize the performance of the RPA solution.

In addition to technical considerations, engineers must also address the human element in the design and development of RPA solutions. They need to focus on creating user-friendly interfaces and intuitive interactions between humans and robots. This includes incorporating proper training and documentation to facilitate seamless collaboration between operators and automated systems.

Ultimately, successful RPA solutions require a holistic approach that encompasses the technical, operational, and human aspects of manufacturing processes. Engineers must continuously strive for excellence by staying updated with the latest advancements in RPA technologies and leveraging their expertise to drive continuous improvement in manufacturing through Robotic Process Automation.

Testing and Deployment of RPA Systems

In the realm of Robotic Process Automation (RPA), engineers play a pivotal role in ensuring the successful testing and deployment of RPA systems. This subchapter delves into the crucial aspects of testing and deployment, providing engineers with key insights and best practices to achieve excellence in the manufacturing industry through RPA.

Testing RPA systems is a critical step in the implementation process. Engineers must conduct rigorous testing to ensure the accuracy, reliability, and efficiency of the automated processes. This involves creating test cases that simulate real-world scenarios and assessing the system's performance against predefined benchmarks. Through thorough testing, engineers can identify and rectify any bottlenecks, errors, or performance issues that may arise during the execution of RPA processes.

One aspect of testing that engineers should pay close attention to is data integrity. RPA systems rely heavily on data inputs and outputs, making it crucial to validate the accuracy and consistency of data throughout the automation process. Engineers should implement data validation checks at different stages of the RPA workflow to ensure that the system is working with accurate and reliable data.

Once the testing phase is complete, engineers must proceed with the deployment of RPA systems. Deployment involves integrating the RPA solution into the existing manufacturing infrastructure, ensuring seamless collaboration between humans and robots. Engineers must carefully plan the deployment strategy, considering factors such as system compatibility, scalability, and potential impact on the workforce.

During the deployment phase, engineers should also focus on monitoring and managing the RPA systems. Continuous monitoring allows engineers to track the performance of the automated processes, identify any anomalies, and make necessary adjustments. Additionally, engineers should establish a robust governance framework to ensure compliance, security, and reliability of the RPA systems.

To achieve excellence in manufacturing through RPA, engineers should also consider the human element. Clear communication and training programs are essential to equip the workforce with the necessary skills to collaborate effectively with the RPA systems. Engineers should facilitate knowledge transfer and provide ongoing support to ensure a smooth transition to the automated environment.

In conclusion, testing and deployment of RPA systems are crucial steps in achieving excellence in manufacturing through Robotic Process Automation. Engineers must employ rigorous testing methodologies, focusing on data integrity and performance evaluation. Additionally, a well-planned deployment strategy and continuous monitoring are vital for successful integration and management of RPA systems. By considering the human element and providing adequate training and support, engineers can ensure a seamless transition to an automated manufacturing environment, unlocking the full potential of RPA.

Continuous Monitoring and Improvement of RPA

In the rapidly evolving landscape of manufacturing, engineers are constantly seeking innovative solutions to enhance productivity and efficiency. One such solution that has gained immense popularity in recent years is Robotic Process Automation (RPA). This subchapter aims to shed light on the crucial aspect of continuous monitoring and improvement of RPA systems, providing engineers in the niche of Robotic Process Automation with valuable insights and strategies to achieve excellence in manufacturing.

Continuous monitoring is an integral part of any successful RPA implementation. It ensures that the automated processes are functioning optimally and meeting the desired objectives. Engineers must establish a robust monitoring framework that includes real-time analytics and reporting capabilities. By monitoring key performance indicators, such as cycle time, error rates, and throughput, engineers can quickly identify bottlenecks and inefficiencies in the RPA system. This allows for timely corrective actions to be taken, ultimately improving process efficiency and reducing downtime.

To facilitate continuous improvement, engineers should leverage the power of data analytics. By collecting and analyzing data from RPA processes, engineers can identify patterns and trends that may go unnoticed otherwise. These insights can be used to optimize the RPA system and make informed decisions regarding process redesign or resource allocation. Additionally, engineers should consider implementing machine learning algorithms that can adapt and improve the RPA system based on real-time data.

Regular audits and assessments are essential to ensure compliance and security in RPA systems. Engineers should conduct periodic audits to evaluate whether the RPA system adheres to industry regulations and organizational policies. Furthermore, security measures such as access controls, encryption, and data segregation should be continuously monitored and updated to mitigate potential risks.

Collaboration between engineers and business stakeholders is vital for the continuous improvement of RPA systems. Regular feedback sessions and brainstorming meetings can foster a culture of innovation and creativity. By involving business stakeholders in the monitoring and improvement processes, engineers can gain valuable insights into the actual business needs and align the RPA system accordingly.

In conclusion, continuous monitoring and improvement of RPA systems are critical for achieving excellence in manufacturing. Engineers must establish a robust monitoring framework, leverage data analytics, conduct regular audits, and collaborate with business stakeholders to optimize the RPA system. By embracing these strategies, engineers in the niche of Robotic Process Automation can drive significant improvements in productivity, efficiency, and overall manufacturing excellence.

Chapter 5: Overcoming Challenges and Pitfalls in RPA Implementation

Addressing Resistance to Change from Workforce

Change is inevitable, especially in the field of manufacturing where advancements in technology are constantly shaping the way we work. One such transformative technology that has gained significant traction in recent years is Robotic Process Automation (RPA). As engineers, it is essential for us to understand the importance of RPA and how it can revolutionize the manufacturing industry. However, introducing RPA into the workforce can be met with resistance, as employees may fear job losses or feel overwhelmed by the prospect of learning new skills. In this subchapter, we will address the resistance to change from the workforce and provide strategies to overcome these challenges.

Firstly, it is important to communicate the benefits of RPA to the workforce. Employees may have misconceptions about RPA replacing human jobs entirely. However, it is essential to emphasize that RPA is designed to automate repetitive and mundane tasks, allowing employees to focus on higher-value activities that require critical thinking and problem-solving skills. By highlighting the potential for increased productivity, improved quality, and reduced human error, employees can see how RPA can enhance their work rather than replace them.

Another effective strategy is involving employees in the transition process. By engaging them in discussions and seeking their input, employees will feel valued and more willing to embrace the change. This can be achieved through training programs, workshops, and interactive sessions that provide the necessary knowledge and skills to work alongside RPA systems. By empowering employees to adapt to new technologies and providing them with opportunities for professional growth, resistance can be minimized.

Additionally, it is crucial to address any concerns or fears that employees may have. Open and transparent communication channels should be established, allowing employees to express their apprehensions and providing reassurance. Highlighting success stories from other organizations that have implemented RPA can also help alleviate fears and build confidence in the process.

Furthermore, creating a supportive work environment is essential for successful implementation. Encouraging collaboration and teamwork between humans and robots can foster a sense of camaraderie and ensure a smooth transition. Recognizing and rewarding employees for their adaptability and contributions to the RPA integration can also boost morale and motivate others to embrace change.

In conclusion, addressing resistance to change from the workforce is crucial when implementing Robotic Process Automation in manufacturing. By effectively communicating the benefits of RPA, involving employees in the transition process, addressing concerns, and creating a supportive work environment, engineers can help facilitate a smooth and successful adoption of RPA. Embracing new technologies like RPA is essential for achieving excellence in manufacturing and staying ahead in today's competitive landscape.

Ensuring Compatibility with Existing Systems and Processes

In the rapidly evolving field of Robotic Process Automation (RPA), one of the key challenges that engineers face is ensuring compatibility with existing systems and processes. As automation technologies continue to advance, it is crucial for engineers to understand how to integrate new robotic processes seamlessly into the existing manufacturing environment. This subchapter aims to provide engineers with valuable insights and strategies to achieve compatibility and maximize the benefits of RPA.

When implementing RPA, engineers must first conduct a comprehensive assessment of the current systems and processes in place. By thoroughly understanding the strengths and weaknesses of the existing infrastructure, engineers can identify areas that could benefit from automation and determine the most suitable robotic processes to implement. This assessment also helps in identifying potential conflicts or bottlenecks that may arise during the integration process.

Compatibility checks are crucial to ensure that the new robotic processes do not disrupt the overall operations. Engineers should carefully analyze the data formats, communication protocols, and interfaces used by the existing systems and processes. This analysis will enable them to design the RPA solutions that seamlessly integrate with the existing infrastructure, minimizing downtime and maximizing efficiency.

Another important aspect of ensuring compatibility is considering the impact of RPA on the workforce. Engineers must collaborate closely with the operations team and the workforce to understand their needs and concerns. By involving the stakeholders throughout the implementation process, engineers can address any resistance, fears, or uncertainties that may arise. This collaborative approach fosters a smooth transition, ensuring that RPA enhances the capabilities of the workforce rather than replacing it.

Furthermore, engineers should pay close attention to the scalability and flexibility of the RPA solutions. As manufacturing processes evolve, the robotic processes must be adaptable to accommodate changes in production volumes, product variations, or emerging technologies. The ability to scale and adjust the RPA solutions easily will ensure the long-term compatibility and effectiveness of the automation systems.

In conclusion, ensuring compatibility with existing systems and processes is a critical aspect of successfully implementing Robotic Process Automation in manufacturing. By conducting a thorough assessment, considering workforce needs, and designing scalable solutions, engineers can ensure seamless integration and maximize the benefits of RPA. This subchapter equips engineers with the knowledge and strategies required to achieve compatibility and excellence in manufacturing through RPA.

Managing Cybersecurity Risks in RPA

In today's digital world, the adoption of Robotic Process Automation (RPA) has become increasingly prevalent in the manufacturing industry. As engineers, it is crucial for us to recognize and address the cybersecurity risks associated with RPA implementation. This subchapter aims to provide an in-depth understanding of the challenges and strategies for managing cybersecurity risks in RPA.

RPA involves the use of software robots to automate repetitive and rule-based tasks, streamlining manufacturing processes and improving operational efficiency. However, with the increasing reliance on interconnected systems and the transfer of sensitive data, a company's cybersecurity becomes a top priority. Cyberattacks can lead to significant financial losses, reputational damage, and even compromise the safety of critical infrastructure.

One of the primary challenges in managing cybersecurity risks in RPA is the complexity of the technology itself. RPA systems often interact with various IT systems and databases, increasing the attack surface for potential threats. Hence, engineers must design and implement robust security measures to protect against unauthorized access, data breaches, and malicious activities.

To mitigate these risks, engineers should prioritize the implementation of a multi-layered security framework. This includes securing RPA infrastructure, establishing strong access controls, encrypting sensitive data, and implementing continuous monitoring and threat detection systems. Regular security audits and penetration testing should also be conducted to identify vulnerabilities and ensure compliance with industry regulations.

Another critical aspect of managing cybersecurity risks in RPA is fostering a culture of cybersecurity awareness among employees. Training programs should be conducted to educate staff on best practices for data protection, identifying phishing attempts, and reporting suspicious activities. Regular communication regarding the importance of cybersecurity and the potential consequences of a breach can significantly reduce the likelihood of human error.

Furthermore, engineers should stay updated with the latest cybersecurity trends and developments. Collaborating with cybersecurity experts and participating in industry forums and conferences can provide valuable insights into emerging threats and best practices for risk management.

In conclusion, managing cybersecurity risks in RPA is a crucial responsibility for engineers in the manufacturing industry. By understanding the challenges and implementing robust security measures, we can safeguard our critical systems, protect sensitive data, and ensure the uninterrupted operation of RPA in manufacturing processes. By adopting a proactive approach and fostering a culture of cybersecurity awareness, we can achieve excellence in manufacturing through the secure implementation of Robotic Process Automation.

Mitigating Potential Ethical and Legal Issues in RPA

As the field of Robotic Process Automation (RPA) continues to advance, engineers must be aware of the potential ethical and legal issues that may arise. While RPA offers numerous benefits, such as increased efficiency and productivity, it also introduces new challenges that need to be addressed to ensure responsible and ethical practices. This subchapter aims to provide engineers in the niche of Robotic Process Automation with valuable insights on mitigating these potential issues.

One of the major ethical concerns surrounding RPA is job displacement. While automation can streamline operations, it also has the potential to replace human workers. Engineers need to consider the impact on the workforce and implement strategies to mitigate job losses. This may include upskilling and reskilling programs to ensure that employees can transition into new roles that complement automation systems. Additionally, engineers should strive to create a work environment that fosters collaboration between humans and robots, emphasizing the unique skills and capabilities of both.

Another ethical consideration is data privacy and security. RPA requires access to sensitive data, and engineers must ensure that proper safeguards are in place to protect this information. Compliance with regulations such as the General Data Protection Regulation (GDPR) should be a top priority. Engineers should implement robust encryption techniques, access controls, and regular audits to minimize the risk of data breaches and ensure the privacy of individuals involved in the automation process.

Moreover, legal issues can arise in the context of RPA. Engineers should be aware of potential intellectual property infringements when utilizing third-party automation solutions. Careful consideration should be given to licensing agreements and intellectual property rights to avoid legal disputes.

Furthermore, engineers must consider potential biases in RPA algorithms. Machine learning algorithms can inadvertently incorporate biases present in the data they are trained on, leading to unfair outcomes or discrimination. Engineers need to regularly monitor and audit algorithms to identify and rectify any biases that may arise.

In conclusion, while Robotic Process Automation offers immense potential for improving manufacturing processes, engineers must be proactive in addressing the ethical and legal challenges associated with it. By mitigating potential job displacement, safeguarding data privacy and security, respecting intellectual property rights, and monitoring for biases, engineers can ensure that RPA is implemented responsibly and ethically. This subchapter serves as a guide for engineers in the niche of Robotic Process Automation, providing them with valuable insights to achieve excellence while maintaining ethical and legal standards.

Paving the Way for Successful RPA Adoption in Manufacturing

Introduction

Robotic Process Automation (RPA) has emerged as a game-changer in the manufacturing industry, revolutionizing the way processes are carried out and offering numerous benefits. This subchapter aims to provide engineers with insights into the successful adoption of RPA in manufacturing and how it can lead to excellence in this field.

Understanding Robotic Process Automation

Robotic Process Automation refers to the use of software robots or virtual workers to automate repetitive and rule-based tasks in manufacturing processes. These intelligent robots are capable of mimicking human actions, such as data entry, data analysis, and decision-making, enabling manufacturers to streamline operations, enhance productivity, and reduce errors.

Identifying the Right Processes for Automation

To ensure successful RPA adoption in manufacturing, engineers need to identify the right processes for automation. This involves analyzing the existing processes, identifying repetitive and rule-based tasks, and assessing their suitability for automation. By selecting the appropriate processes, engineers can maximize the benefits of RPA and achieve operational excellence.

Ensuring Compatibility and Integration

Before implementing RPA in manufacturing, engineers must ensure compatibility and integration with existing systems and technologies. This includes assessing the compatibility of the RPA software with the manufacturing software and hardware infrastructure. Seamless integration is essential to ensure smooth operations, data flow, and communication between the RPA system and other manufacturing systems.

Designing and Developing RPA Solutions

Engineers play a crucial role in designing and developing RPA solutions tailored to the specific manufacturing requirements. This involves mapping out the automation process, configuring the software robots, and developing the necessary scripts and algorithms. Engineers must consider factors such as process complexity, scalability, and security while building RPA solutions.

Training and Collaboration

Successful RPA adoption in manufacturing requires training and collaboration among engineers and other stakeholders. Engineers should provide comprehensive training to employees on how to work alongside software robots and utilize the automation tools effectively. Collaboration between engineers, process owners, and IT departments is also crucial to ensure a smooth transition and address any challenges that may arise during the implementation phase.

Measuring and Optimizing RPA Performance

To achieve excellence in manufacturing through RPA, engineers must continuously measure and optimize the performance of the automation system. This involves tracking key performance indicators (KPIs), such as cycle time reduction, error rate, and cost savings. Engineers should analyze the data obtained from the RPA system and identify areas for improvement to enhance productivity and efficiency further.

Conclusion

Robotic Process Automation has the potential to revolutionize manufacturing by streamlining processes, enhancing productivity, and reducing errors. For engineers, successful RPA adoption requires careful consideration of process selection, compatibility, integration, designing and development, training, collaboration, and performance optimization. By paving the way for successful RPA adoption in manufacturing, engineers can achieve excellence in this field and drive the industry forward.

Chapter 6: Training and Skill Development for RPA Engineers

Key Skills and Competencies Required for RPA Engineers

In today's rapidly evolving world of manufacturing, Robotic Process Automation (RPA) has emerged as a game-changing technology. RPA engineers play a crucial role in designing, implementing, and maintaining automated systems that streamline manufacturing processes. To excel in this field, engineers need to possess a unique set of skills and competencies that enable them to navigate the complexities of RPA effectively.

First and foremost, RPA engineers must have a solid foundation in engineering principles. They should be well-versed in mechanical, electrical, and software engineering to understand the intricacies of automated systems. A strong grasp of mathematics and physics is essential to design and optimize robotic processes. Additionally, knowledge of programming languages such as Python, Java, or C++ is crucial for developing and customizing RPA solutions.

Furthermore, RPA engineers should have a deep understanding of manufacturing processes. They must be able to analyze existing workflows and identify areas where automation can add value. By applying their expertise, RPA engineers can optimize manufacturing operations, reduce human error, and enhance productivity. Familiarity with Lean and Six Sigma methodologies is highly beneficial as it allows engineers to identify waste and implement lean automation solutions.

Another critical skill for RPA engineers is problem-solving. They must be able to identify bottlenecks, troubleshoot issues, and devise creative solutions. RPA engineers often encounter technical challenges that require critical thinking and analytical skills. The ability to think outside the box and find innovative ways to overcome obstacles is essential for success in this field.

Strong communication and collaboration skills are also vital for RPA engineers. They often work in multidisciplinary teams, including software developers, electrical engineers, and manufacturing experts. Effective communication ensures smooth collaboration and a shared understanding of project goals. RPA engineers must be able to translate complex technical concepts into clear and concise language for non-technical stakeholders.

Lastly, RPA engineers must possess a passion for continuous learning and staying up-to-date with the latest advancements in the field. RPA is a rapidly evolving technology, and engineers need to adapt to new tools, techniques, and best practices. They should actively seek out training opportunities, attend conferences, and engage in professional networking to stay at the forefront of RPA innovation.

In conclusion, RPA engineers play a crucial role in achieving excellence in manufacturing through Robotic Process Automation. By possessing a strong foundation in engineering principles, a deep understanding of manufacturing processes, problem-solving skills, effective communication, and a passion for continuous learning, engineers can excel in the niche of RPA.

Training Programs and Certifications for RPA Engineers

In the fast-paced world of Robotic Process Automation (RPA), staying ahead of the curve is essential for engineers to excel in their careers. As the demand for RPA engineers continues to rise, it becomes crucial to acquire the necessary skills and certifications to stand out in this competitive field. This subchapter will explore various training programs and certifications available to engineers seeking excellence in manufacturing through RPA.

Training programs for RPA engineers provide a comprehensive understanding of the concepts, tools, and techniques required for successful implementation of automation processes. These programs cover various aspects such as process mapping, workflow design, software integration, and data analysis. One popular training program is offered by the Robotic Industries Association (RIA), which provides a thorough overview of RPA technologies and their applications in manufacturing. The RIA training program equips engineers with the knowledge and skills needed to develop, deploy, and maintain RPA systems effectively.

Certifications validate an engineer's expertise in RPA and enhance their professional credibility. The UiPath Certified RPA Developer certification is widely recognized in the industry and demonstrates proficiency in building and deploying RPA solutions using the UiPath platform. Another notable certification is the Automation Anywhere Certified Advanced RPA Professional, which validates an engineer's ability to design and develop complex RPA workflows. These certifications not only showcase an engineer's technical skills but also serve as a valuable asset for career advancement and job opportunities in the rapidly growing RPA market.

Beyond general RPA training programs and certifications, engineers can also specialize in specific RPA niches. For instance, those interested in the healthcare sector can pursue training programs that focus on RPA applications in healthcare operations and patient data management. Similarly, engineers interested in finance can explore programs tailored to RPA solutions for financial processes such as invoice processing, fraud detection, and compliance.

In conclusion, training programs and certifications play a pivotal role in the professional development of RPA engineers. By investing in these learning opportunities, engineers can gain a competitive edge in the field of Robotic Process Automation. Whether it is through comprehensive training programs provided by organizations like the RIA or industry-recognized certifications such as UiPath Certified RPA Developer, these resources enable engineers to stay up-to-date with the latest advancements and best practices in RPA. Specialized training programs also allow engineers to target specific niches, expanding their expertise and opening doors to exciting opportunities in various industries. As the demand for RPA engineers continues to grow, continuous learning and certification will be crucial in achieving excellence in manufacturing through Robotic Process Automation.

Continuous Learning and Professional Development in RPA

In the ever-evolving field of Robotic Process Automation (RPA), engineers play a vital role in driving innovation, efficiency, and excellence in manufacturing processes. As the demand for automation continues to grow, it is crucial for engineers to embrace continuous learning and professional development to stay at the forefront of this dynamic industry.

Continuous learning is not just a buzzword; it is a necessity in the world of RPA. With technology advancing rapidly, engineers must constantly update their knowledge and skills to remain competitive. The subchapter "Continuous Learning and Professional Development in RPA" aims to provide insights and guidance on how engineers can enhance their expertise and contribute to the advancement of the field.

One of the key aspects of continuous learning is staying abreast of the latest trends and developments in RPA. Engineers should actively seek out educational resources, attend conferences, and join professional networks to stay connected with the industry's pulse. By immersing themselves in the RPA community, engineers can gain valuable insights, engage in meaningful discussions, and develop a deeper understanding of the challenges and opportunities in their niche.

Professional development is another crucial component for engineers in the RPA field. This subchapter will explore various avenues for professional growth, including certifications, training programs, and workshops. By investing in their professional development, engineers can acquire new skills, expand their knowledge base, and enhance their problem-solving abilities. These efforts not only benefit individuals but also contribute to the advancement of the RPA industry as a whole.

Furthermore, the subchapter will address the importance of cross-disciplinary learning. RPA is a multidisciplinary field that requires expertise in engineering, computer science, data analytics, and more. Engineers should actively collaborate with professionals from different disciplines to gain a holistic understanding of RPA and its applications. By embracing a diverse and collaborative approach, engineers can leverage their collective knowledge and drive innovation in manufacturing processes.

In conclusion, continuous learning and professional development are vital for engineers in the niche of Robotic Process Automation. By staying updated with the latest trends, actively pursuing professional development opportunities, and embracing cross-disciplinary learning, engineers can achieve excellence in manufacturing through RPA. This subchapter serves as a guide for engineers to enhance their skills, expand their knowledge, and contribute to the advancement of the RPA industry.

Collaboration and Knowledge Sharing in the RPA Community

In the rapidly evolving field of Robotic Process Automation (RPA), engineers play a critical role in driving innovation and achieving excellence in manufacturing. As the RPA community continues to grow, collaboration and knowledge sharing become essential for engineers to stay at the forefront of this transformative technology.

Collaboration within the RPA community allows engineers to pool their expertise, experiences, and insights. By working together, they can tackle complex challenges, share best practices, and develop innovative solutions. Through collaboration, engineers can leverage each other's strengths, learn from one another's mistakes, and accelerate the pace of progress in RPA implementation.

One of the primary avenues for collaboration in the RPA community is through forums and online communities. These platforms provide a space for engineers to connect with their peers, ask questions, and engage in discussions. By actively participating in these forums, engineers can tap into a wealth of collective knowledge, gain new perspectives, and explore different approaches to problem-solving. The power of collaboration in these online communities lies in the diversity of voices and experiences, enabling engineers to think beyond their individual limitations and push the boundaries of what is possible.

Furthermore, knowledge sharing plays a crucial role in advancing the field of RPA. Engineers must not only collaborate but also actively contribute to the community by sharing their own insights and experiences. By documenting their successes and failures, engineers can create a repository of knowledge that future generations can build upon. This shared knowledge becomes a valuable resource for engineers facing similar challenges, allowing them to learn from past projects and avoid reinventing the wheel. Additionally, engineers can contribute to the RPA community by publishing research papers, presenting at conferences, and conducting workshops, further disseminating their expertise and findings.

To foster collaboration and knowledge sharing, it is essential for engineers in the RPA community to embrace a culture of openness and continuous learning. They must be willing to share their knowledge, seek help when needed, and remain receptive to new ideas. Engaging in mentorship programs, attending industry conferences, and participating in training workshops are also effective ways for engineers to expand their networks, learn from industry experts, and stay up to date with the latest trends in RPA.

In conclusion, collaboration and knowledge sharing are vital components of achieving excellence in manufacturing through Robotic Process Automation. By actively participating in the RPA community, engineers can collaborate, learn from each other, and collectively drive the adoption and advancement of RPA technology. Embracing a culture of openness and continuous learning will not only benefit individual engineers but also contribute to the overall growth and success of the RPA community.

Chapter 7: Case Studies: Successful RPA Implementations in Manufacturing

Case Study 1: RPA in Automotive Manufacturing

Introduction

The integration of Robotic Process Automation (RPA) has revolutionized the manufacturing industry, and the automotive sector is no exception. This case study explores the application of RPA in automotive manufacturing, highlighting its benefits, challenges, and potential solutions. Addressing engineers and those interested in robotic process automation, this chapter aims to provide valuable insights into how RPA has enhanced efficiency, productivity, and overall performance in the automotive manufacturing niche.

Benefits of RPA in Automotive Manufacturing

RPA has transformed the automotive manufacturing landscape by streamlining various processes and improving overall productivity. By automating repetitive and mundane tasks, engineers can focus on more critical aspects, such as design and innovation. RPA has significantly reduced human error and increased accuracy, resulting in improved product quality and customer satisfaction. Additionally, RPA has optimized supply chain management, enhancing inventory control, and minimizing delays.

Case Study: Implementation of RPA in an Automotive Assembly Line

This case study delves into a real-life example of RPA implementation within an automotive assembly line. The objective was to automate the production process, reduce costs, and enhance operational efficiency. Engineers analyzed the existing manual tasks, such as component installation, quality control, and documentation, and identified areas suitable for automation.

Through the integration of RPA, robots were deployed to handle repetitive tasks, reducing the need for human intervention. This not only improved efficiency but also decreased the risk of injuries in hazardous environments. The robots were programmed to perform tasks accurately, resulting in higher product quality and reduced defects. Furthermore, data collection during the production process was automated, enabling real-time monitoring and analysis, leading to data-driven decision making.

Challenges and Solutions

While the implementation of RPA in automotive manufacturing brings numerous benefits, certain challenges must be addressed. Engineers faced resistance from some employees who feared job displacement. However, by emphasizing the transition towards more complex and fulfilling roles, the workforce was gradually reassigned to positions that required higher skill levels.

Another challenge was the integration of RPA with existing legacy systems and machinery. Engineers had to ensure compatibility and develop comprehensive training programs for seamless transition and adoption. Additionally, the security of sensitive data and protection against potential cyber threats were critical concerns that required robust measures and regular updates.

Conclusion

This case study aimed to showcase the successful implementation of RPA in automotive manufacturing. By automating repetitive tasks, engineers can focus on more complex and innovative aspects, leading to improved productivity, enhanced product quality, and reduced costs. While challenges exist, such as employee resistance and system integration, proactive measures and comprehensive training programs can help overcome them. RPA has undoubtedly revolutionized the automotive manufacturing niche, and engineers must continue to embrace this technology to achieve excellence in their respective fields.

Case Study 2: RPA in Electronics Manufacturing

Introduction:
In this subchapter, we will delve into a fascinating case study that highlights the application of Robotic Process Automation (RPA) in the electronics manufacturing industry. As engineers, it is crucial to understand how RPA can revolutionize and optimize processes within this niche. Let's explore the various ways in which RPA has reshaped electronics manufacturing, leading to enhanced productivity, efficiency, and cost savings.

Background:
The electronics manufacturing industry is known for its high-speed production lines, intricate assembly processes, and complex quality control measures. These factors create a fertile ground for RPA implementation. By deploying software robots, engineers can automate repetitive tasks, reduce human errors, and streamline production workflows.

Case   Study:
In this case study, we will focus on a leading electronics manufacturer that faced challenges in optimizing their assembly line. This company integrated RPA into their production processes to address these issues and achieve excellence in manufacturing.

1.   Automating   Component   Inspection:
One of the primary applications of RPA in electronics manufacturing is automating component inspection. By leveraging computer vision technologies, software robots can quickly and accurately identify faulty or misplaced components. This significantly reduces the need for manual inspection, saves time, and ensures high-quality products.

2. Streamlining Inventory Management: RPA also plays a pivotal role in streamlining inventory management processes. By connecting with the company's Enterprise Resource Planning (ERP) system, software robots can automatically track inventory levels, generate purchase orders when supplies are running low, and update stock records in real-time. This automation eliminates the need for manual data entry, reduces errors, and minimizes inventory holding costs.

3. Enhancing Production Planning: With RPA, engineers can optimize production planning by automating the generation and adjustment of production schedules. By considering various factors such as demand forecasts, machine availability, and workforce capacity, software robots can create optimized schedules that maximize productivity and minimize downtime.

4. Improving Quality Control: RPA can revolutionize quality control processes by automating the inspection and testing of finished products. Software robots can perform comprehensive tests, record results, and compare them against predefined quality standards. This automation ensures that only defect-free products reach the market, enhancing customer satisfaction and brand reputation.

Conclusion:
The case study presented here demonstrates the immense potential of RPA in revolutionizing electronics manufacturing. By leveraging software robots, engineers can achieve excellence in manufacturing through improved component inspection, streamlined inventory management, enhanced production planning, and superior quality

control. As engineers, it is crucial to embrace RPA as a tool that can transform the electronics manufacturing industry, paving the way for increased efficiency, reduced costs, and improved competitiveness.

Case Study 3: RPA in Pharmaceutical Manufacturing

Introduction:
In this case study, we will explore the application of Robotic Process Automation (RPA) in the pharmaceutical manufacturing industry. RPA has emerged as a game-changing technology that has revolutionized various sectors, and the pharmaceutical industry is no exception. As engineers specializing in Robotic Process Automation, it is crucial for us to understand the challenges faced by pharmaceutical manufacturers and how RPA can help overcome them.

Challenges in Pharmaceutical Manufacturing: Pharmaceutical manufacturing involves complex processes, stringent regulations, and a constant need for quality control. Traditional manufacturing methods often suffer from inefficiencies, human errors, and the risk of contamination. Engineers face the challenge of streamlining these processes while ensuring compliance with regulatory standards. This is where RPA comes into play.

RPA Benefits in Pharmaceutical Manufacturing: Robotic Process Automation offers numerous benefits in the pharmaceutical manufacturing industry. Firstly, it enhances operational efficiency by automating repetitive tasks such as data entry, report generation, and inventory management. This not only reduces the workload on human workers but also minimizes the chances of errors.

Secondly, RPA improves compliance with regulatory standards. The software robots can be programmed to follow strict protocols, ensuring that every step of the manufacturing process adheres to regulatory requirements. This significantly reduces the risk of non-compliance and potential penalties.

Another advantage of RPA in pharmaceutical manufacturing is the ability to integrate and analyze vast amounts of data. By extracting data from various sources, RPA systems can generate real-time insights, enabling engineers to make data-driven decisions for process optimization and continuous improvement.

Case Study: Implementing RPA in a Pharmaceutical Manufacturing Facility:

Let us now delve into a real-life case study where RPA was successfully implemented in a pharmaceutical manufacturing facility. By automating data collection from laboratory instruments, inventory management, and quality control processes, the facility achieved significant cost savings, increased accuracy, and enhanced productivity.

The case study will provide a detailed analysis of the implementation process, challenges faced, and the positive outcomes achieved through RPA. It will serve as a practical guide for engineers in the pharmaceutical industry who are contemplating the adoption of RPA.

Conclusion:

Robotic Process Automation has become a powerful tool for engineers in the pharmaceutical manufacturing industry. By automating repetitive tasks, ensuring compliance, and harnessing the power of data analysis, RPA enables manufacturers to achieve excellence in their operations. This case study highlights the benefits and challenges of implementing RPA in pharmaceutical manufacturing, providing valuable insights for engineers in this niche of Robotic Process Automation.

Lessons Learned from Successful RPA Implementations

Robotic Process Automation (RPA) has emerged as a game-changer in the manufacturing industry, revolutionizing the way engineers approach repetitive and time-consuming tasks. As engineers continue to explore the potential of RPA, it is crucial to learn from successful implementations to ensure the highest level of excellence in manufacturing. This subchapter aims to highlight key lessons learned from successful RPA implementations, providing engineers with valuable insights and tips to enhance their own automation projects.

Lesson 1: Define Clear Objectives

One of the most critical lessons from successful RPA implementations is the importance of defining clear objectives from the outset. Engineers must identify the specific tasks and processes they aim to automate and establish measurable goals. Defining objectives helps create a roadmap for the implementation and ensures that the automation aligns with the broader manufacturing goals.

Lesson 2: Collaborate Across Teams

Successful RPA implementations emphasize the need for collaboration across various teams, including engineers, process owners, IT experts, and operators. By involving all stakeholders throughout the implementation process, engineers can gain valuable insights, address concerns, and foster a culture of innovation. Collaboration fosters a shared understanding of the automation's potential and encourages a sense of ownership among the key players.

Lesson 3: Prioritize Process Optimization

RPA implementations should not solely focus on automating existing processes but also prioritize process optimization. Engineers must carefully analyze and streamline processes before automation to eliminate unnecessary steps and inefficiencies. By optimizing processes beforehand, engineers can ensure that RPA is integrated seamlessly, maximizing its effectiveness and efficiency.

Lesson 4: Continuous Improvement

Successful RPA implementations recognize the importance of continuous improvement. Engineers should constantly monitor and evaluate the performance of the automated processes, identifying areas of improvement and implementing necessary adjustments. By adopting an iterative approach, engineers can enhance the automation's capabilities, adapt to changing manufacturing needs, and drive excellence in the long run.

Lesson 5: Training and Support

Training and support play a crucial role in the success of RPA implementations. Engineers must provide adequate training to the end-users, ensuring they understand the benefits and functionalities of the automated processes. Ongoing support and assistance should be readily available to address any challenges or concerns that may arise, ensuring a smooth transition to RPA.

In conclusion, learning from successful RPA implementations is essential for engineers seeking excellence in manufacturing through Robotic Process Automation. By defining clear objectives, collaborating across teams, prioritizing process optimization, embracing continuous improvement, and providing training and support, engineers can unlock the true potential of RPA. Each lesson learned contributes to creating a foundation for successful RPA implementations, empowering engineers to transform manufacturing processes and achieve unparalleled excellence.

Insights and Best Practices for Future RPA Projects

Introduction

As engineers in the field of Robotic Process Automation (RPA), it is crucial to stay ahead of the curve by continuously seeking insights and adopting best practices for future projects. This subchapter aims to provide valuable guidance to engineers in the RPA niche, helping them achieve excellence in manufacturing through the implementation of RPA. By incorporating these insights and best practices into their projects, engineers can enhance efficiency, productivity, and overall operational effectiveness.

Understanding the evolving landscape
To excel in RPA projects, engineers must stay up-to-date with the latest developments in the field. This involves understanding emerging technologies, such as machine learning and artificial intelligence, and their potential applications in RPA. By keeping a pulse on the evolving landscape, engineers can identify new opportunities and leverage cutting-edge solutions to optimize manufacturing processes.

Designing scalable RPA solutions
One of the key challenges in RPA projects is scalability. Engineers must design solutions that can be easily expanded or modified to accommodate future requirements. This necessitates a modular approach to RPA implementation, where components can be added or removed as needed. By designing scalable RPA solutions, engineers can ensure long-term effectiveness and adaptability, saving time and resources in the future.

Effective process analysis and optimization
Before implementing RPA, engineers must thoroughly analyze existing processes and identify areas for improvement. This involves

conducting detailed process mapping, identifying bottlenecks, and streamlining workflows. By optimizing processes prior to RPA implementation, engineers can maximize the benefits of automation and minimize any potential disruptions.

Ensuring data security and compliance

Data security and compliance are paramount in RPA projects, especially in manufacturing where sensitive information is often involved. Engineers must prioritize implementing robust security measures and ensuring compliance with industry regulations. This includes encryption, access controls, and regular audits to safeguard data integrity and protect against cyber threats.

Continuous monitoring and improvement

Once RPA solutions are implemented, engineers should establish a framework for continuous monitoring and improvement. Regular performance analysis and data-driven insights can help identify areas for optimization and fine-tuning. By fostering a culture of continuous improvement, engineers can ensure that RPA projects remain relevant and effective in the long run.

Conclusion

In summary, achieving excellence in manufacturing through RPA requires engineers to stay updated on the latest trends and technologies, design scalable solutions, optimize processes, ensure data security and compliance, and establish a framework for continuous monitoring and improvement. By adopting these insights and best practices, engineers can pave the way for successful RPA projects and drive manufacturing excellence in their respective industries.

Chapter 8: Future Trends and Innovations in RPA for Manufacturing

The Role of Artificial Intelligence and Machine Learning in RPA

As engineers in the field of Robotic Process Automation (RPA), it is crucial for us to understand the evolving role of Artificial Intelligence (AI) and Machine Learning (ML) in driving innovation and efficiency. In this subchapter, we will explore the significant impact of AI and ML on RPA and how they contribute to achieving excellence in manufacturing processes.

AI and ML technologies have revolutionized the way we approach RPA. Traditionally, RPA systems were designed to automate repetitive and rule-based tasks, mimicking human actions. However, with the integration of AI and ML, RPA systems are now capable of advanced cognitive tasks, decision-making, and self-improvement.

One of the most valuable contributions of AI and ML to RPA is their ability to process and analyze vast amounts of data. Manufacturing processes generate enormous volumes of data, and AI and ML algorithms can extract meaningful insights from this data, enabling engineers to optimize processes, identify bottlenecks, and make data-driven decisions.

AI also plays a crucial role in enhancing the accuracy and reliability of RPA systems. Through natural language processing and computer vision, AI-powered robots can interpret and understand unstructured data, such as documents, images, and videos, with remarkable precision. This capability allows engineers to automate tasks that previously required human intervention, reducing errors and improving overall process efficiency.

Machine Learning, on the other hand, empowers RPA systems to continuously learn and adapt. By analyzing historical data and patterns, ML algorithms can identify anomalies and predict future outcomes. This predictive capability enables engineers to proactively address potential issues, optimize production schedules, and improve resource allocation, ultimately leading to enhanced productivity and cost savings.

Furthermore, AI and ML enable RPA systems to interact and collaborate with humans more effectively. Natural language processing and sentiment analysis algorithms enable robots to understand and respond to human inputs, making human-robot collaboration seamless and intuitive. This human-like interaction fosters a more productive and efficient work environment, where engineers can focus on higher-value tasks while allowing the RPA systems to handle routine and repetitive tasks.

In conclusion, the integration of AI and ML in RPA has transformed the manufacturing landscape by enabling advanced cognitive abilities, data-driven decision-making, and improved collaboration between humans and robots. As engineers, it is essential for us to embrace these technologies and leverage their potential to achieve excellence in manufacturing processes. By harnessing AI and ML, we can drive innovation, optimize operations, and unlock new levels of productivity in the world of Robotic Process Automation.

Collaborative Robots (Cobots) and Human-Robot Interaction

In recent years, the field of Robotic Process Automation (RPA) has witnessed remarkable advancements, with Collaborative Robots (Cobots) emerging as a prominent subset. Cobots are revolutionizing the manufacturing industry by transforming the way humans and robots interact in the workplace. This subchapter delves into the intricacies of Cobots and their impact on Human-Robot Interaction (HRI), providing engineers in the niche of Robotic Process Automation with invaluable insights.

Unlike traditional industrial robots that operate in isolation, Cobots are designed to work alongside humans, enhancing productivity, efficiency, and safety on the factory floor. HRI, therefore, plays a crucial role in ensuring seamless collaboration between humans and Cobots. Engineers working in RPA must understand the various factors that influence HRI and the key considerations for successful implementation.

One of the primary concerns in HRI is safety. Collaborative robots are equipped with advanced sensors and actuators that enable them to detect the presence of humans and modify their behavior accordingly. This ensures that the Cobots operate at a reduced speed or stop completely when a human enters their workspace. Engineers need to carefully analyze the safety requirements and standards specific to their manufacturing environment to ensure that Cobots are integrated safely and effectively.

Another crucial aspect of HRI is ergonomics. Cobots are designed to assist humans in physically demanding tasks, alleviating the risk of musculoskeletal injuries. Engineers need to consider the ergonomic needs of the operators, ensuring that the Cobots are easy to operate, intuitive, and adapt to the workflow seamlessly. User-centered design principles and usability testing play a vital role in optimizing the interaction between humans and Cobots.

Furthermore, communication and collaboration are key elements in successful HRI. Engineers need to explore the various methods of communication between humans and Cobots, such as visual cues, voice commands, and touch interfaces. Effective communication channels facilitate efficient task allocation, error handling, and problem-solving, enhancing the overall productivity of the manufacturing process.

In conclusion, the emergence of Collaborative Robots (Cobots) has transformed the landscape of Robotic Process Automation, emphasizing the importance of Human-Robot Interaction (HRI). Engineers working in the niche of RPA must understand the intricacies of HRI to successfully integrate Cobots into manufacturing processes. Safety, ergonomics, and communication are crucial considerations, ensuring that Cobots work seamlessly alongside humans, enhancing productivity, efficiency, and safety in the manufacturing industry.

Integration of RPA with Internet of Things (IoT) in Manufacturing

In recent years, the manufacturing industry has witnessed significant advancements in technology, particularly in the areas of Robotic Process Automation (RPA) and the Internet of Things (IoT). These innovations have revolutionized the way factories operate, leading to improved efficiency, productivity, and cost-effectiveness. This subchapter explores the integration of RPA with IoT in the manufacturing sector, highlighting the benefits, challenges, and future prospects for engineers specializing in Robotic Process Automation.

The integration of RPA with IoT in manufacturing holds immense potential for streamlining and optimizing various processes. RPA involves the use of software robots to automate repetitive tasks, while IoT connects physical devices and machines using sensors and data communication networks. By combining these two technologies, engineers can create a seamless and interconnected system that enhances productivity and minimizes human intervention.

One of the key advantages of integrating RPA with IoT is the ability to collect real-time data from various machines and devices on the factory floor. This data can be analyzed to identify patterns, predict maintenance requirements, and optimize production schedules. For instance, sensors embedded in machines can transmit data on parameters such as temperature, pressure, and speed to the RPA system. The software robots can then analyze this data and make informed decisions regarding maintenance or process adjustments, ensuring smooth operations and preventing costly breakdowns.

Furthermore, the integration of RPA with IoT can enable engineers to monitor and control manufacturing processes remotely. Through a centralized control system, engineers can access real-time data and remotely operate machines and equipment. This not only reduces the need for physical presence on the shop floor but also allows for quick response times in case of any anomalies or emergencies.

However, the integration of RPA with IoT also presents challenges that engineers must overcome. One of the major challenges is ensuring the security and privacy of data transmitted between devices and the RPA system. With the increasing interconnectivity of devices, the risk of cyberattacks and data breaches also increases. Engineers need to implement robust security measures to safeguard sensitive information and ensure the integrity of the system.

In conclusion, the integration of RPA with IoT in manufacturing offers a multitude of benefits for engineers specializing in Robotic Process Automation. By leveraging real-time data and automation capabilities, engineers can optimize production processes, enhance efficiency, and reduce costs. However, it is essential to address the challenges associated with security and privacy to ensure the successful implementation of this integration in the manufacturing sector. As technology continues to evolve, engineers must stay abreast of the latest developments in RPA and IoT to achieve excellence in manufacturing.

Industry 4.0 and Smart Manufacturing: Implications for RPA

In recent years, the manufacturing industry has witnessed a paradigm shift with the emergence of Industry 4.0 and the widespread adoption of smart manufacturing technologies. These advancements have revolutionized the way factories operate, enabling increased efficiency, productivity, and flexibility. One technology that plays a crucial role in this transformation is Robotic Process Automation (RPA).

RPA refers to the use of software robots or "bots" to automate repetitive and rule-based tasks that were traditionally performed by humans. It has already gained significant traction in various industries, including manufacturing, due to its ability to streamline processes, reduce errors, and improve overall operational efficiency. However, with the advent of Industry 4.0 and smart manufacturing, the implications for RPA are even more profound.

One of the key aspects of Industry 4.0 is the integration of cyber-physical systems, the Internet of Things (IoT), and cloud computing. These technologies enable real-time data collection, analysis, and communication, providing manufacturers with valuable insights into their operations. RPA can leverage this wealth of data to make more informed decisions and optimize processes further. For example, by analyzing real-time production data, RPA can automatically adjust manufacturing parameters to ensure optimal efficiency and quality.

Moreover, smart manufacturing emphasizes the concept of interconnectedness, where machines, systems, and humans collaborate seamlessly. RPA can play a vital role in this collaborative environment by acting as a bridge between disparate systems and enabling smooth data exchange. This ensures that critical information flows seamlessly across the production floor, allowing for faster decision-making and improved coordination between different stakeholders.

Another significant implication of Industry 4.0 for RPA is the increased focus on customization and personalization. As consumer demands become more diversified, manufacturers need to adapt quickly and efficiently. RPA can enable this agility by automating the customization process, from order processing to production, reducing lead times and costs associated with customization.

In conclusion, Industry 4.0 and smart manufacturing have profound implications for Robotic Process Automation in the manufacturing industry. RPA can leverage real-time data, facilitate seamless data exchange, and enable customization and personalization, leading to increased efficiency and competitiveness. As engineers in the niche of Robotic Process Automation, it is crucial to understand these implications and harness the power of RPA to achieve excellence in manufacturing in this new era of Industry 4.0 and smart manufacturing.

Predictions for the Future of RPA in Manufacturing

The realm of manufacturing is undergoing a significant transformation with the integration of Robotic Process Automation (RPA). As engineers, it is essential to recognize the potential impact and embrace the opportunities that RPA brings to the table. In this subchapter, we will explore some predictions for the future of RPA in manufacturing, shedding light on how it will revolutionize various niches within the industry.

1. Increased Efficiency and Productivity: RPA holds the promise of streamlining repetitive and mundane tasks, enabling engineers to focus on more complex and strategic activities. As the technology advances, we can expect RPA to become more sophisticated, leading to improved efficiency, reduced errors, and increased overall productivity within manufacturing processes.

2. Collaborative Robots: The emergence of collaborative robots, or cobots, will revolutionize the manufacturing landscape. Cobots are designed to work alongside human operators, enhancing their capabilities and augmenting their skills. With the integration of RPA, these cobots can perform repetitive tasks with precision and accuracy, freeing up human workers to engage in more creative and cognitive activities.

3. Enhanced Quality Control: RPA can play a crucial role in ensuring stringent quality control standards in manufacturing. By automating inspection processes, RPA can detect defects, inconsistencies, and deviations from specifications more effectively than human operators. This will lead to a significant reduction in defective products, minimizing waste and improving overall customer satisfaction.

4. Supply Chain Optimization: RPA has the potential to transform supply chain management within the manufacturing sector. By automating inventory management, order processing, and logistics, RPA can optimize the flow of materials, reduce lead times, and improve the efficiency of the entire supply chain. This will result in cost savings, improved customer service, and a competitive edge for manufacturers.

5. Predictive Maintenance: RPA combined with artificial intelligence can enable predictive maintenance in manufacturing plants. By continuously monitoring equipment and analyzing data in real-time, RPA can forecast potential breakdowns, enabling proactive maintenance actions. This will minimize downtime, extend the lifespan of machinery, and reduce maintenance costs.

6. Adaptability and Scalability: RPA is incredibly adaptable and scalable, making it suitable for a wide range of manufacturing processes and industries. As technology advances, we can expect RPA solutions to become more affordable, user-friendly, and customizable. This will enable manufacturers to adopt RPA at various stages of their production lines, from small-scale operations to large-scale factories.

In conclusion, the future of RPA in manufacturing looks promising for engineers. By embracing this transformative technology, we can expect increased efficiency, improved quality control, optimized supply chains, and enhanced productivity. As engineers, it is crucial to stay informed about the latest advancements in RPA and harness its potential to achieve excellence in manufacturing.

Chapter 9: Conclusion and Final Thoughts

Recap of Key Concepts and Insights

In this subchapter, we will take a moment to recap the key concepts and insights discussed throughout the book "Achieving Excellence in Manufacturing through Robotic Process Automation: An Engineer's Perspective." This recap is particularly relevant to engineers who specialize in the field of Robotic Process Automation (RPA) and are seeking to enhance their knowledge and understanding of this rapidly evolving technology.

Throughout the book, we have explored various aspects of RPA and its applications in the manufacturing industry. We began by providing a comprehensive introduction to RPA, highlighting its potential to revolutionize traditional manufacturing processes. We discussed the benefits of implementing RPA, including increased productivity, improved quality control, and reduced costs.

One of the key themes that emerged was the importance of integrating RPA with existing manufacturing systems. We emphasized the need for engineers to thoroughly understand the manufacturing processes and identify areas where RPA can be effectively deployed. By seamlessly integrating robots into the existing workflow, engineers can optimize production and achieve higher levels of efficiency.

The book also delved into the various types of robots used in RPA, such as collaborative robots (cobots) and industrial robots. We discussed their capabilities, limitations, and suitability for different manufacturing tasks. Understanding the strengths and weaknesses of each type of robot is crucial for engineers to make informed decisions when selecting the most appropriate solution for their specific needs.

Additionally, we explored the challenges and considerations associated with implementing RPA in a manufacturing environment. From safety concerns to programming complexities, engineers must navigate several factors to ensure a successful deployment. We provided valuable insights and practical tips to address these challenges and mitigate potential risks.

Furthermore, we highlighted the importance of continuous learning and staying updated with the latest advancements in RPA. As engineers, it is essential to embrace a mindset of lifelong learning and actively seek opportunities to expand our knowledge base. This can be achieved through attending conferences, participating in workshops, and engaging in online forums dedicated to RPA.

In conclusion, this subchapter served as a recap of the key concepts and insights discussed throughout the book. It reinforced the importance of integrating RPA into manufacturing processes, understanding different types of robots, addressing implementation challenges, and embracing continuous learning. Engineers specializing in RPA can utilize these key takeaways to further enhance their expertise and contribute to achieving excellence in manufacturing through Robotic Process Automation.

The Importance of RPA in Driving Manufacturing Excellence

In today's fast-paced world, where efficiency and productivity are paramount, the manufacturing industry is constantly seeking ways to stay ahead of the competition. One powerful tool that has emerged in recent years is Robotic Process Automation (RPA). In this subchapter, we will explore the significance of RPA in driving manufacturing excellence and its impact on the engineering community.

RPA, as a technology, refers to the use of software robots to automate repetitive and rule-based tasks in manufacturing processes. These robots are capable of mimicking human behavior, allowing them to perform tasks with precision, accuracy, and speed. By implementing RPA in manufacturing operations, engineers can streamline and optimize various processes, achieving higher levels of efficiency, cost reduction, and overall excellence.

One key advantage of RPA in manufacturing is its ability to enhance process automation. By automating tasks such as data entry, inventory management, and quality control, engineers can eliminate human errors, reduce process lead times, and improve overall product quality. This results in increased productivity, reduced operational costs, and improved customer satisfaction.

Moreover, RPA enables engineers to focus on higher-value tasks that require critical thinking and problem-solving skills. By delegating repetitive and mundane tasks to robots, engineers can concentrate on more strategic activities, such as process improvement, innovation, and enhancing product design. This not only enhances job satisfaction but also leads to continuous improvement and innovation within the manufacturing industry.

Furthermore, RPA can enhance collaboration and communication among engineers and other stakeholders. By automating data collection, analysis, and reporting, RPA facilitates real-time access to accurate information, enabling faster decision-making and effective collaboration. This leads to improved coordination among different teams, resulting in enhanced overall operational efficiency and manufacturing excellence.

In conclusion, Robotic Process Automation (RPA) plays a pivotal role in driving manufacturing excellence. By automating repetitive tasks, RPA enhances process efficiency, reduces costs, and improves product quality. It empowers engineers by freeing them from mundane tasks, allowing them to focus on higher-value activities and driving innovation. Moreover, RPA fosters collaboration and communication among different stakeholders, leading to improved coordination and overall operational excellence. As engineers, embracing RPA as a valuable tool is crucial for staying competitive in the ever-evolving manufacturing landscape.

Closing Remarks and Encouragement for Future RPA Endeavors

As we come to the end of this book, I would like to take a moment to reflect on the incredible journey we have embarked upon together. Throughout the preceding chapters, we have explored the fascinating world of Robotic Process Automation (RPA) from an engineer's perspective, delving into the intricacies and possibilities that this technology holds for the manufacturing industry. Now, as we conclude our discussion, I want to leave you with some closing remarks and encouragement for your future RPA endeavors.

First and foremost, I want to commend you, my fellow engineers, for your dedication and passion in seeking excellence in manufacturing through RPA. The decision to embrace automation in our processes is not an easy one, and it requires a deep understanding of our industry and the potential impact of RPA. By choosing to be at the forefront of this technological revolution, you have already proven yourselves as visionaries and pioneers.

Throughout this book, we have discussed the various benefits that RPA brings to the manufacturing industry, including increased efficiency, improved quality control, and enhanced safety. However, it is crucial to remember that RPA is not a one-size-fits-all solution. Each manufacturing process is unique, and it is our responsibility as engineers to analyze, optimize, and adapt RPA to suit the specific needs of our organizations.

As you move forward in your RPA endeavors, I encourage you to foster a culture of innovation and collaboration within your teams. RPA is not just about implementing a new technology; it is about transforming the way we work and collaborate. By involving all stakeholders, from operators to managers, in the decision-making process, we can ensure a smooth transition and maximize the benefits that RPA brings.

Furthermore, I urge you to stay updated with the latest advancements in RPA and related technologies. This field is continuously evolving, and new opportunities and challenges will arise. By staying informed and continuously learning, we can adapt and leverage these advancements to further excel in our manufacturing processes.

In conclusion, I want to emphasize that RPA has the potential to revolutionize the manufacturing industry. By embracing this technology and harnessing its power, we can achieve unprecedented levels of excellence in our processes. I am confident that as engineers, you have the skills, knowledge, and determination to lead the way in this transformative journey. Let us embrace RPA wholeheartedly, collaborate passionately, and continue to push the boundaries of what is possible. Together, we can achieve excellence in manufacturing through Robotic Process Automation.